Fatty Liver Diet Cookbook

100 Recipes To Fight Fatty Liver Disease And Live Longer

Eileen Fisher

DEDICATION

To my sisters, Faye and Stella. Your support went a long way!

TABLE OF CONTENT

INTRODUCTION

The Liver is the second largest gland in the body and the only organ that can regenerate when healthy. It helps in various way like storing, processing, detoxifying, and transporting nutrients, toxic, and medication substances into the blood. It supports in filtering any harmful thing in the system, absorbing important nutrient to the body, indigestion, and in blood clotting.

So many people are having issues with their health and can be traceable to their diet or what they take in that leads to fatty liver disease also known as hepatic steatosis. Fats in the liver cannot be harmful except in excess, this is very dangerous and can lead to liver inflammation. Taking a lot of heavy drinks too store up fats and affect the liver in functioning appropriately. But this disease can occur even without taking alcohol.

Types Of Fatty Liver Disease

There are two types of fatty liver disease:

• Non Alcoholic Fatty Liver Disease (NAFLD)

This type can be classified into two;

The simple Non Alcoholic Fatty Liver disease – occurs to people that don't take alcohol and no inflammation in the liver but fat is excess through insulin resistance, high triglycerides or overweight. And it can be reversible or get worse.

Non Alcoholic Steatohepatitis (NASH) – occurs to people that don't take alcohol too but it's more serious, the liver cells are damaged and there is inflammation in the liver. Can lead to cancer, fibrosis, or cirrhosis.

Non Alcoholic Fatty Liver and Non Alcoholic steatohepatitis diseases existence are unknown but can be caused by wrong food intake or genes.

• <u>Alcoholic Fatty Liver Disease (AFLD)</u>

This is the earliest stage, also known as alcohol hepatitis. This is caused by too much of alcohol, and excess fat which can inflame the liver, damage the liver cells and stop the liver to function as it's should. But can be prevented by taking of no alcohol.

Cause Of Fatty Liver Disease

Fatty liver disease occur when the liver cannot metabolize fat any more, occur through some specific genes, side effects of some drugs used, age–the older you get, and by diversities of things such as:

• Excess alcohol

• High blood sugar

• Speedy weight loss

• High level of cholesterol

• Obesity

• Malnourished

• Hepatitis C

• Exposure to certain toxins

• Pregnancy complications

Symptoms Of Fatty Liver Disease

Sometimes symptoms are not noticeable but some people may have symptoms like;

• Weakness

• Itchy skin

• Red palm

• Nausea

• Nose bleeding

• Yellowish skin and eyes

• Dark patches on the skin

• Fatigue

• Weight loss

• Swelling of legs

• Abdominal pain and swelling

• Drowsiness

How To Reverse Fatty Liver Disease

<u>Lose Weight And Exercise</u>

Regardless of the type of fatty liver disease you re diagnosed with you need to lose weight to aid reduction of inflammation, scarring and fat in the liver. If possible, if you're overweight, you should be ready to lose at least 10 percent of your body weight gradually not at a time because losing of weight at a time is dangerous to the body. Exercise will help you lose weight as necessary and reduce fat, garlic oil helps in losing of weight too. You exchange carbohydrates to energy instead of fat while exercising. Maintaining regularly exercise will go a long way, it's not compulsorily severe ones. It's just required that your heart pump not for body building.

<u>Follow Healthy Diet</u>

To reverse fatty liver disease you need to develop the habit of eating healthy foods. Take more protein, avoid excess calories, cut down carbs, and sustain a plant base diet. Take lot of fresh fruits, vegetables, sea foods and lean meat. You also need to quit taking heavy drinks, it will only get worse and lead to more serious liver disease if not stopped.

Healthy foods that you need are:

Nuts And Seeds

Nuts and seed contain antioxidant, vitamins, good source or of glutathione, and omega-3 acid that helps the liver to function well. Vitamin C and E stops the advancing of fatty liver disease. Such as walnut, sunflower seeds, Brazil nut, almonds, Chai-seeds, flaxseeds and lot more.

Citrus and beetroot also contain vitamin C.

Fruits And Vegetables

This are antioxidants that fight against inflammation, reduces fat in the liver and provides vitamins and minerals that makes liver function well. Such as avocado, spinach, blueberry, horseradish, papaya, kale, raspberry, citrus fruits, arugula, grape, broccoli, Brussel sprout, cauliflower, asparagus, cabbage, watercress, tomatoes, cherries and collards.

Whole Grain, And Legumes

Such as kidney beans, brown rice, lentils, black beans, sweet potatoes, quinoa, oat, peanuts, green peas, whole grain bread and pasta, navy beans, pinto beans, bulgur, and more.

Flour based food (cakes, breads, snacks, and more), and processed foods are bad for this diet but unprocessed or slightly processed whole grain is best for this diet because it helps in reducing cholesterol.

Sea Foods, Lean Meats, And Fatty Fish

Promote you liver health with fatty fish such as tuna, trout, salmon, and lot more. Also animal foods like chicken, egg, turkey and more.

Fat in fatty fish improves insulin resistance and reduce fat intensely.

Healthy Fats

Monounsaturated fats is best for this diet, it improves liver enzymes and improves blood levels. Such as oil from nuts, olive oil, coconut oil, flaxseed oil, canola oil, avocado oil, and lot more. Also avoid animal fats.

Coffee

This is the best drink for a healthy liver, reduces risk of cirrhosis, inflammation, the danger of increasing liver disease, and reduces symptoms of liver disease.

Taking of tea, either black or green tea goes a long way too, so healthy because it also helps in reduction of cholesterol, and assist liver function.

Supplements

This may provide direct nourishment straight to the liver.

Glutathione

Curcumin

Green Tea Extract

Garlic oil

Carnitine

Zinc and Selenium

Following this diet as well as the recipes in this book, will not only reduce fatty liver, but help reduce symptoms and make you stay healthy.

Welcome to a healthy living!

BREAKFAST RECIPES

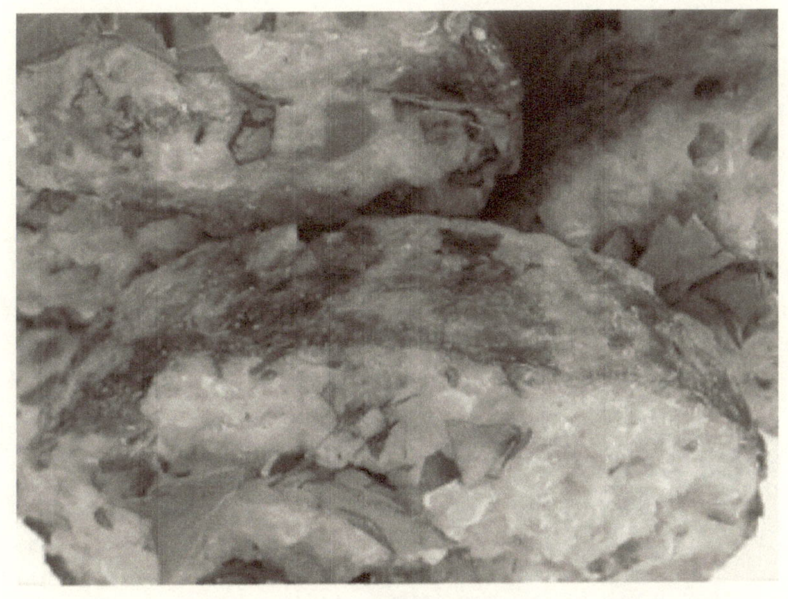

Quiche Cups
Beat this up with any veggies of your choice for you breakfast. So tasty!

Serves: 6

<u>Ingredients</u>

2 eggs

¼ cup dried tomato, chopped

3 egg whites

¼ cup leek, chopped

10ounce kale, chopped

¼ cup yellow bell pepper, seeded & chopped

<u>Directions</u>

1. Mix egg, egg whites, tomatoes, bell pepper, leek, and kale together in a bowl. Line and spray six muffin cups and put mixture in each cups.

2. Then preheat the oven to 350°F and bake.

Beet and Potato Egg Basket
The taste is super and it is healthy too!

Serves: 1

<u>Ingredients</u>

2 tablespoons red beet, peeled an shredded

2 tablespoons hash brown potatoes, shredded

2eggs

Pepper

<u>Directions</u>

1. Mix all ingredient together except the eggs and pepper, share into two halves.

2. Put in muffin cup and bake until soft then break one egg on each muffin then bake for about 15 minutes. Sprinkle pepper and enjoy!

Healthy Oatmeal Breakfast

Classic and enjoyable!

Serves: 1

<u>Ingredients</u>

½ cup steel rolled oats, cooked

1 teaspoon pure maple syrup

1 teaspoon honey

<u>Directions</u>

1. Mix all ingredients together and enjoy!

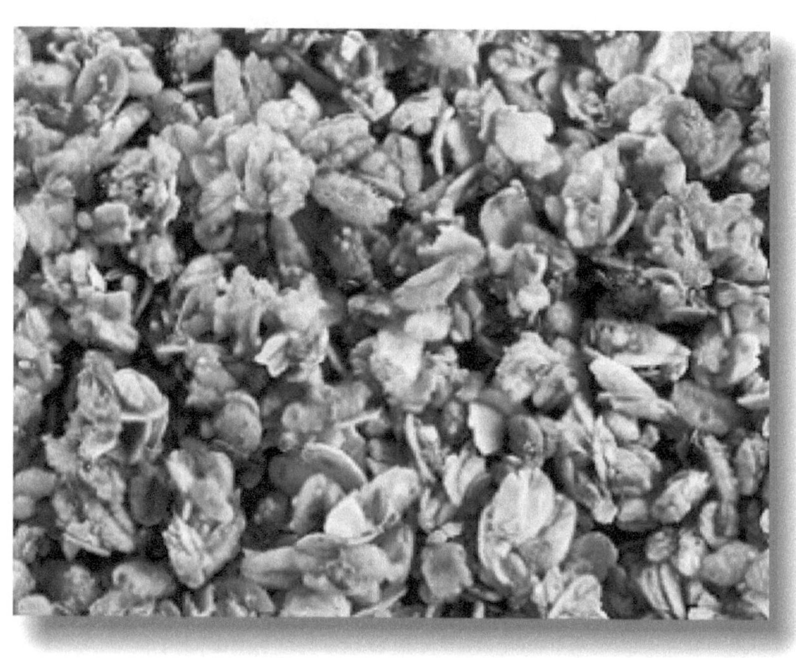

Honey Granola

You need to taste this!

Serves: 3

Ingredients

4 cups rolled oats

1 cup golden raisins

2 cups nuts, chopped

2 teaspoons ground cinnamon

3/4 cup honey

1 teaspoon vanilla extract

1/2 cup butter

1/4 teaspoon salt

Directions

1. Mix nuts, raisins, and oats in a bowl. Then combine and boil separately, cinnamon, butter, vanilla, honey and salt in a pan on medium heat.

2. Put honey mixture in it and stir. Put in a cookie sheet already greased and spread evenly.

3. Bake in an oven at 350 degrees for about 30 minutes. When ready let it cool, and crumble.

Zucchini, Herb and Potato Egg Basket
This will go well for breakfast!

Serves: 1

Ingredients

2 tablespoons zucchini, shredded

1 teaspoon flat-leaf parsley, chopped

2 tablespoons shredded brown potatoes

1/2 teaspoon fresh chives, chopped

2eggs

Pepper

Directions

1. Mix all ingredients together except the eggs and pepper, share into two halves. Put in muffins cup and bake until soft then break one egg on each muffin and bake for about 15 minutes. Sprinkle pepper and enjoy!

Buffalo Chicken Sandwich
A g4ood way to start your day

Serves: 8

Ingredients

8 oz. Chicken breast (boneless skinless), cooked and also shredded

2 tablespoon butter, heated

1/2 cup Frank's Red Hot

1/4 tablespoon black pepper

2 tablespoon vinegar

Directions

1. Mix all ingredients in a bowl and bake for about 30 minutes at 350 degree. Enjoy!

Mini Vegetable Frittatas
This is healthy for you!

Serves: 9

Ingredients

2 tablespoon low-fat milk

2 cups broccoli, chopped

2 oz. goat cheese, pounded

1 cup diced tomato

5 eggs, whisked

Salt

Pepper

Directions

1. Mix all ingredients together in a bowl, add salt and pepper to taste and put mixture in muffin tins already sprayed. Bake at 350 degree for about 15 minutes. Enjoy!

Baked Egg Cups

Super nutritious!

Serves: 6

Ingredients

1/2 cup cheddar cheese, shredded

Lean deli ham6 slices

1 tablespoon chopped chives

6 eggs

Pepper

Directions

1. Lay a ham slice each in six cups of muffin sprayed and bake for about 10 minutes at 350 degree.

2. Break one egg in each cup and sprinkle pepper and bake again for about 10 minutes too. Serve!

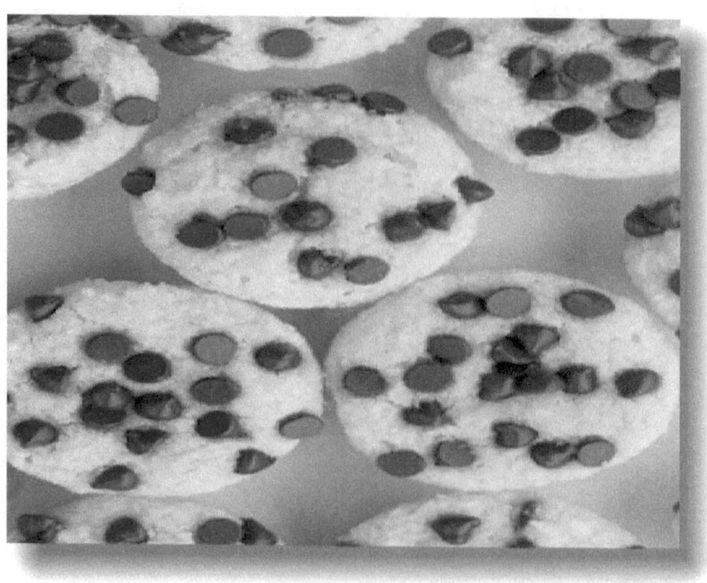

Applesauce Oatmeal Muffins

So tasty!

Serves: 12

Ingredients

1/2 cup unsweetened applesauce

1 cup whole wheat flour

1 cup old fashioned oats, soaked in skim milk

1 teaspoon baking powder

1/2 teaspoon baking soda

1/2 cup brown sugar

1 teaspoon cinnamon

2 egg whites

1 teaspoon sugar

1/2 teaspoon salt

Directions

1. Spray muffin with cooking spray. Mix all ingredient together in a bowl and make sure it is well combined.

2. Bake for about 25 minutes at 400 degree. Enjoy when cool!

Non-Dairy Cornmeal Breakfast
Really tasty!

Serves: 1

Ingredients

1½ cups unsweetened almond milk

2 cups cold water

1 cup corn meal

2 cups cold water

Grape seed oil

Pure maple syrup

Salt

Directions

1. Heat up almond milk powder in a saucepan, add corn meal and stir well.

2. When it is thick, turn down heat, add grape seed oil, syrup, and salt. Enjoy!

Potato Egg Basket
This will make your breakfast!

Serves: 2

Ingredients

1/4 cup brown potatoes, shredded

Pepper

2eggs

Directions

1. Share potatoes into two and put in muffin cup, bake for few minutes or until soft then break one egg on each muffin cup and bake for about 15 minutes.

2. Sprinkle pepper and serve.

Oatmeal Breakfast

You will definitely enjoy this!

Serves: 1

Ingredients

½ cup steel rolled oats, cooked

1 teaspoon ground cinnamon.

½ cup fist full of raisins

1 teaspoon pure maple syrup

1 teaspoon clover honey

1 cup water

Directions

1. Add all ingredients in a bowl and mix well. Enjoy!

Gluten-Free Blueberry Banana Pancakes

Serves: 1

Ingredients

1½ ripe bananas, peeled and mashed

½ cup fresh blueberries

1/8 teaspoon baking powder

2 large eggs, whisked

Directions

1. Add all ingredients together except fresh blueberries and mix well. In a sauté pan sprayed with cooking spray on medium heat, put batter.

2. Sprinkle fresh blueberries and flip to the other side to cook. Serve.

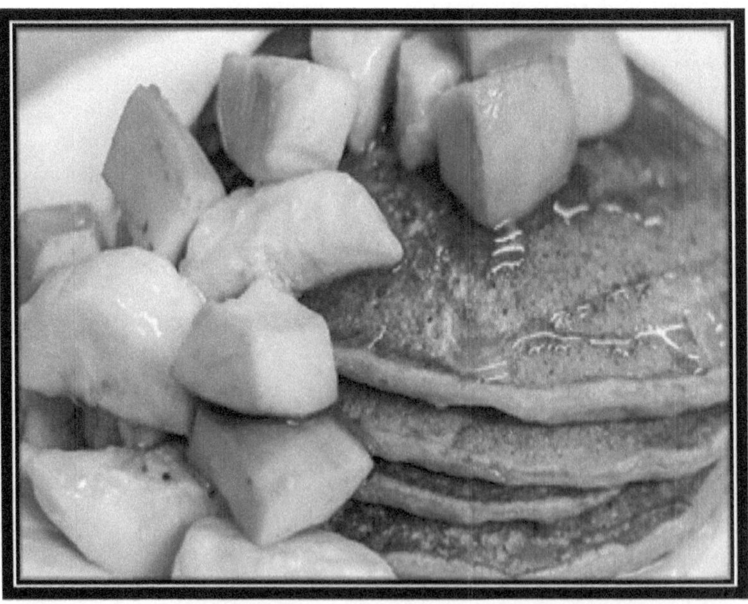

Carrot and Potato Egg Basket

Sweet! You should try this!

Serves: 1

Ingredients

2 tablespoons refrigerated shredded hash brown potatoes

2 tablespoons shredded carrot

2eggs

Pepper

Directions

1. Mix carrot and potatoes together and share into two halves.

2. Put in muffin cup and bake until soft then break one egg on each muffin and bake for about 15 minutes. Sprinkle pepper and enjoy!

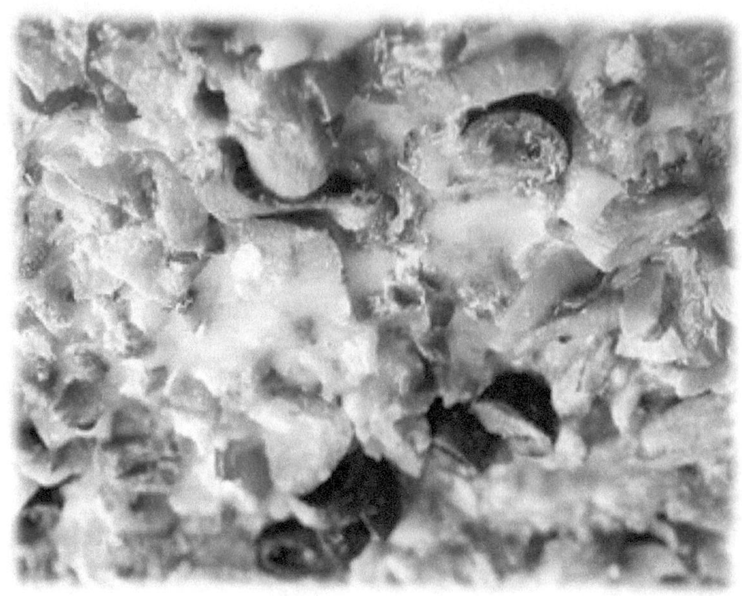

Grilled Cheese Pizza Sandwich
Yummy! You should taste this.

Serves: 1

<u>Ingredients</u>

1 teaspoon Parmesan, shredded

2 tablespoons marinara sauce

1/4 cup mozzarella cheese

2 slices mixed grain bread

Salt

Pepper

Directions

1. On each bread spread marina sauce, mozzarella cheese, and sprinkle parmesan cheese. Sauce side down too

2. Put the bread together and straight into the heated pan. Let the cheese melt and outside is brown. Enjoy!

Mini Eggplant Pizzas

You should have this for breakfast.

Serves: 1

Ingredients

1 eggplant, cut into 4 slices

1/2 cup part-skim mozzarella cheese, shredded

1/4 cup pasta sauce

4 teaspoons olive oil

1/8 teaspoon ground black pepper

1/2 teaspoon salt

Directions

1. Brush both sides with oil and add salt and pepper. Bake for about 8 minutes at 425 degrees till brown.

2. Then put pasta sauce and shredded cheese on them, bake until cheese is melted and enjoy.

Asian Chicken Salad

Sumptuous!

Serves: 1

Ingredients

2 cups chicken, skinned, cooked, and cut

1 cucumber, cut

1 mandarin orange, divided

4 cups cabbage, shredded

2 tablespoons cilantro, chopped

1/2 cup nonfat Asian dressing

1 cup mushrooms, cut

1 cup carrots, grated

3 green onions, cut

Black pepper

Directions

1. Mix mushrooms, cabbage, carrots, chicken, cucumber, dressing, and cilantro in a large bowl. Add pepper to taste and garnish with tangerine and onions.

Taco Soup

Healthy and tasty for you!

Serves: 6

Ingredients

16 ounces extra lean ground beef

1 tomatoes and green chilies, diced

½ cup chickpeas, drained and mashed

1 dark kidney beans, drained

1 cup canned corn kernels

1 recipe Taco Seasoning

1 can tomato sauce, no salt

1 yellow onion, chopped

Directions

1. In a large sauce pan, fry ground beef and onion on medium heat, put seasoning, tomato sauce, kidney beans, diced tomato and water.

2. Simmer for 10 minutes and put corn and chickpeas. Enjoy when ready.

Deviled Eggs
You need this for lunch.

Serves: 6

Ingredients

3 tablespoons mayonnaise, fat free

1 teaspoon dill pickle, chopped

1 teaspoon Dijon mustard

1 tablespoon celery, chopped fine

1/4 teaspoon black pepper

1 tablespoon parsley, chopped

1 teaspoon pickle juice

6 boiled eggs, cut into half

Directions

1. Mash only yolks and add all ingredient, stir well and toss in to egg halves.

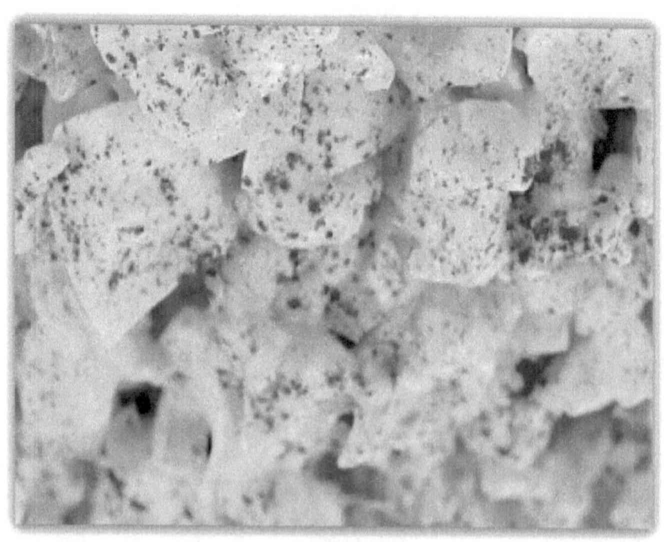

Eggplant Stew

Yummy! This stew is filling!

Serves: 10

Ingredients

1 eggplant, cut in cubes

3 summer squash, sliced

8 oz. sliced mushrooms

4 zucchini, sliced

1 teaspoon crushed garlic

1 can of diced tomatoes

1 large onion, chopped

1 tablespoon olive oil

Salt and pepper to taste

Directions

1. Cook onion and garlic with oil for about 10 minutes, put mushrooms and tomatoes.

2. Then add eggplant, and simmer for about 45 minutes, put squash, zucchini, chickpeas and spices. Enjoy when vegetables are ready.

Roasted Corn and Pepper Soup
Great meal you need to taste!

Serves: 8

Ingredients

4 yellow corn, shucked

16 oz. vegetable broth, low sodium

1 tablespoon olive oil

¼ teaspoon cumin, ground

3 bell peppers

1 ½ cups diced tomatoes, drained

1/2 teaspoon dried thyme

1/4 teaspoon black pepper

1 yellow onion, diced

¼ red pepper

Directions

1. Bake at 400 degree corn and peppers, remove kernels from cob and remove core and charred skin from pepper.

2. Chop peppers, add oil to pan, cook onions, and ingredients. Simmer for about 20 minutes.

3. Blend in an immersion blender and enjoy.

Best Tuna Salad

Delicious salad ever!

Serves: 8

Ingredients

1 can tuna, drained

1/2 Fuji apple, chopped

2 tablespoon fat free miracle

1/3 cup dried cranberries

Romaine lettuce, for topping

1 onion, chopped

Salt

Directions

1. Add all ingredients in a bowl, mix well, put lettuce in a plate and top with the mixture. Enjoy!

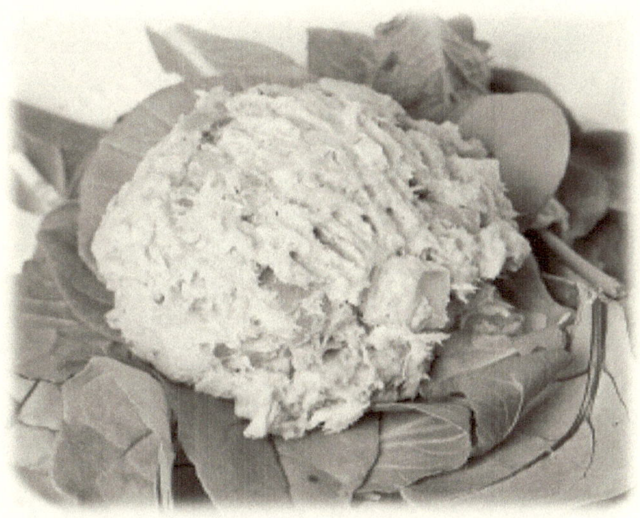

Low-Carb Lettuce Wraps

Juicy and well flavored!

Serves: 1

Ingredients

3.5 ounces lean ground beef

1 clove garlic, crushed

1/4 garlic powder

1/4 dried oregano

1 tablespoon onion, minced

Cayenne pepper to taste

Chopped cilantro to taste

1/4 onion powder

Salt and black pepper to taste

Directions

1. When beef is brown, put garlic, onion, spices and water. Cook for about 10 minutes. Add pepper and salt to taste. Enjoy!

Layered Mexican Dip with Baked Lime Chips

Super easy and tasty too!

Serves: 6

Ingredients

2 whole-wheat tortillas, sliced

1 lime, cut in half

1 cup fat-free Greek yogurt

1 tablespoon taco seasoning

14.5 oz. fat-free refried beans

1/2 cup black beans, rinsed

1 tablespoon cilantro, chopped

1/4 cup reduced-fat cheese, shredded

1/2 avocado, chopped

2 Roma tomatoes, diced

1 cup green leaf lettuce, shredded

3 green onions, chopped

1/8 teaspoon salt

Directions

1. Put tortillas on baking sheet, spray with cooking spray and put salt. Bake at 350 degrees until crispy for about 5 minutes.

2. Add juiced half of lime and put avocado and cilantro in it, put seasoning and the second half of lime together, yogurt and refrigerate for a while.

3. Stir refried beans, black beans, cheese, green onions, and yogurt mixture. Top with lettuce avocado and tomatoes.

Lean Philly Cheese Steak

This sandwich is for you. Enjoy!

Serves: 1

Ingredients

2 ounces extra lean roast beef, cooked and sliced

1 oz. provolone

1/4 teaspoon dried thyme

1/2 whole wheat pita pocket

1/4 teaspoon black pepper, cracked

½ cup mushrooms, sliced

1 onion, sliced

Directions

1. Warm skillet on medium heat, coat with cooking spray, put mushrooms, thyme, onion, and pepper. Cook for about 5 minutes.

2. Put water and stir. Add meat, and cheese. When cheese melts remove from heat and use to fill the wheat pita pocket. Serve and enjoy!

Chilled Vegetable Soup

Easy and tasty soup! You will definitely ask for more.

Serves: 6

Ingredients

1 slice whole grain bakery bread, crust away and bite-size pieced

1 red pepper, seeds away and chopped

1-2 tablespoons red wine vinegar

1 cucumber, peeled and cut

1 banana pepper, seeds away and cut

1/2 teaspoon black pepper

5 large tomatoes

2 cloves garlic

1/2 onion, chopped

Directions

1. Put bread and water in bowl, cover for about 5 minutes. Blend in a food processor peppers, garlic, cucumber, onions and tomatoes.

2. Drain water from bread and add to the pepper mixture, process for about 20 seconds. Put pepper and vinegar to taste well.

3. Garnish with diced avocado and enjoy!

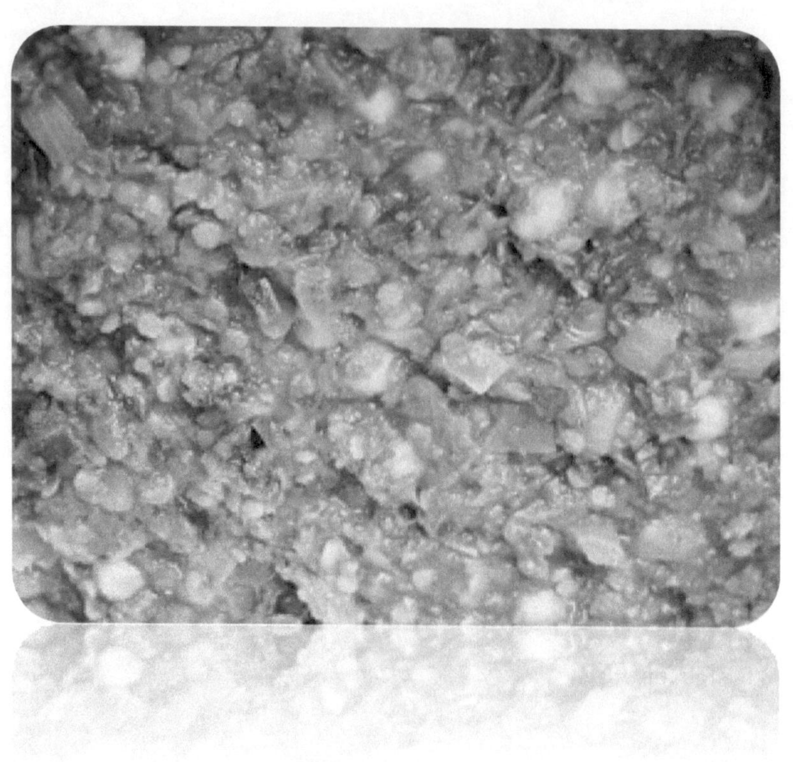

Taco Style Lentils and Brown Rice
So easy and delicious too!

Serves: 4

<u>Ingredients</u>

3/4 cup brown rice, not cooked

3/4 cup dry lentils

4 cups beef broth

1 tsp. cumin

1/2 tsp. garlic powder

1 tbsp. chili powder

1 tsp. onion powder

<u>Directions</u>

1. Put all ingredients in a pot and boil for about 35 minutes. Make sure the water is absorbed or dried. Enjoy!

DINNER RECIPES

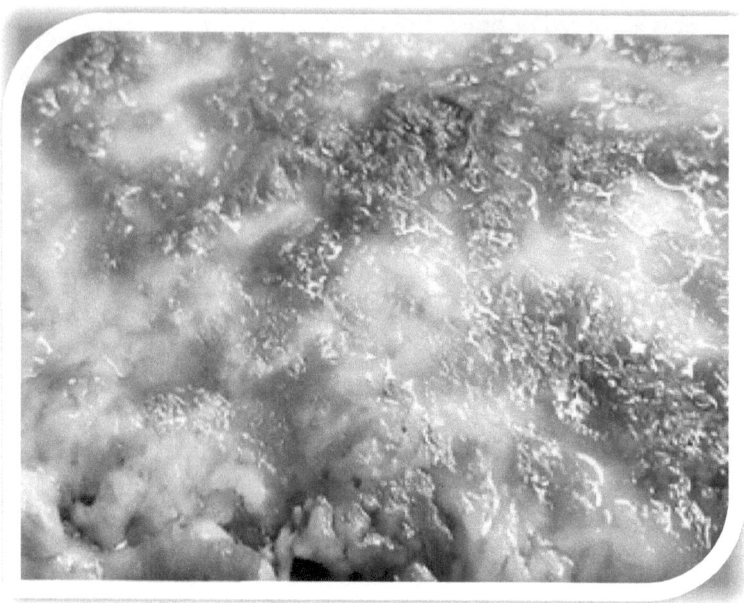

Skillet Lasagna
Tasty and best for dinner!

Serves: 6

Ingredients

1 pound lean ground beef

1 tablespoon dried parsley flakes

1 teaspoon dried basil leaves

2 ½ cups whole wheat lasagna noodles, broken-up

1 cup fat-free cottage cheese

1/4 cup fat-free Parmesan cheese, grated

1 small onion, chopped

3 cloves garlic, minced

8 ounces tomato sauce

1 can diced tomatoes

1 egg

1 ¼ cups water

1 teaspoon dried oregano leaves

1 teaspoon salt

Directions

1. Brown beef, add onions, garlic, tomatoes, tomato sauce, oregano, parsley, basil, and water.

2. Add pasta and simmer for about 20 minutes, mix cheeses, egg, basil and pepper in a bowl and add to pasta mixture cook for about 5 minutes.

3. Top with shredded mozzarella and enjoy!

Slow Cooker Marinara Chicken and Vegetables

Yummy! You will like this!

Serves: 8

Ingredients

2 pounds chicken breasts, boneless and skinless

1 bell pepper, seeded, and diced

2 zucchini, diced

18-ounce jar low-sodium marinara sauce

1 teaspoon dried basil

4 tomatoes, chopped

1 teaspoon dried thyme

4 cloves garlic, crushed

4 ribs celery, diced

Directions

1. In a slow cooker, put chicken, tomatoes, zucchini, garlic, celery, sauce, and pepper.

2. Add basil and thyme and set slow cooker on low and cook for about 7 hours. Enjoy!

Slow Cooker Lasagna

Best for your dinner!

Serves: 8

<u>Ingredients</u>

6 lasagna noodles

1 pound ground beef, lean

24-ounce jar marinara sauce, low-sodium

2 cups pound eggplant, diced

1 cup cheese blend, shredded

1 tablespoon fresh parsley, chopped

1/4 teaspoon red pepper flakes

15 ounces part-skim ricotta cheese

2 teaspoon dried thyme

¼ cup egg substitute

<u>Directions</u>

1. Brown beef, add red pepper flakes, sauce, water, thyme, and eggplant. Add small portion of meat sauce to slow cooker.

2. Mix cheese, ricotta, parsley, and egg substitute in a bowl and add to the meat sauce in the slow cooker. Then add the remaining meat sauce.

3. Set slow cooker and cook for 4 hours.

Spicy Taco Soup

Hearty for your consumption!

Serves: 8

Ingredients

1 lb. ground beef

2 cans pinto beans

1 can black beans

1 package ranch style dressing mix

1 can cream-style corn

1 package taco seasoning

2 cans diced tomatoes with green chilies

1 onion, chopped

Directions

1. Brown beef and add all ingredients. Add water if needed and cook for about 20 minutes. Enjoy!

Mexican Chicken and Rice Casserole

You will love it more!

Serves: 12

Ingredients

1 1/2 cup instant rice

1 can fat free cream chicken soup

1 can fat free cream mushroom soup

1 can black beans, and rinsed

1 can tomatoes with chilies, diced

1 tablespoon taco seasoning

3 pounds chicken breasts, boneless and skinless

1 cup cheddar cheese, shredded

Directions

1. Mix soups, seasoning, and water together in a bowl. Spray a dish and add mixture. Add rice, chicken breast, tomatoes, beans, onions and cilantro.

2. Use foil to cover dish and bake at 350 for about 1 hour or more. Sprinkle cheese and bake for about 10 minutes. Serve!

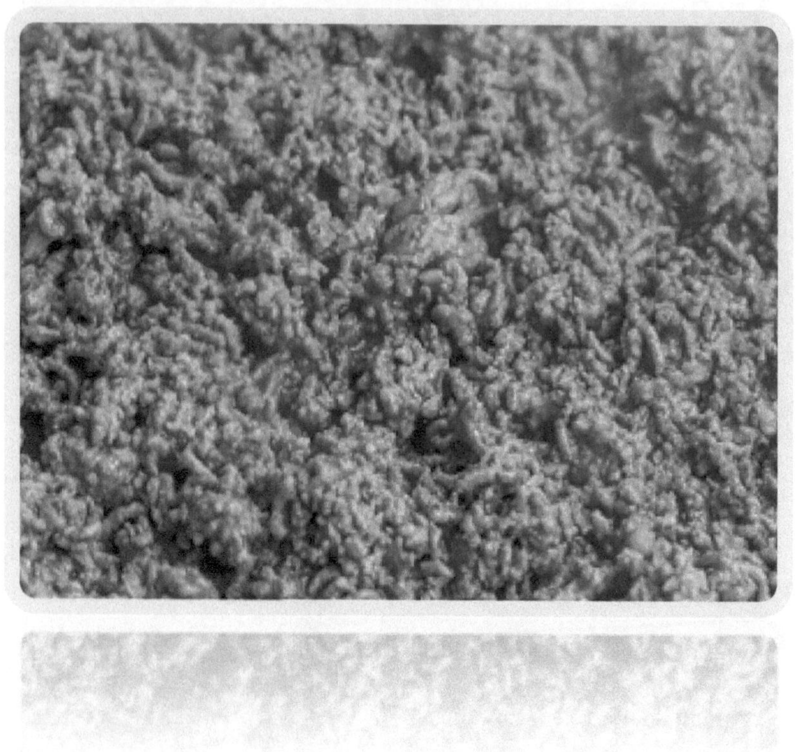

Ground Beef Casserole

Super easy and tasty!

Serves: 6

<u>Ingredients</u>

1.5 lbs. lean ground sirloin

1 cup potatoes, diced

2 cups canned, crushed tomatoes

1 cup frozen peas

1/2 teaspoon cinnamon

1/2 teaspoon ginger

1 tablespoon curry powder

1/2 teaspoon turmeric

1 cup onions, chopped

Salt and pepper to taste

Directions

1. Brown sirloin, add onions, peas, spices, tomatoes, potatoes, salt and pepper.

2. Cook for about 25 minutes. Serve and enjoy!

Beef and Broccoli

Hearty and tasty! You need this for your dinner.

Serves: 4

Ingredients

1 lb. round steak, sliced

4 cups rice, cooked

1 can beef broth

2 tablespoon cornstarch

2 tablespoon soy sauce

1 tablespoon brown sugar

1/4 teaspoon ground ginger

4 cups broccoli florets

1/4 teaspoon garlic powder

1 clove garlic, minced

1/2 cup onion, chopped

Directions

1. After spraying your skillet with cooking spray, put onion, beef, and garlic on medium heat to brown. Set aside.

2. Simmer half of broth and broccoli in a pan until soft, mix the remaining ingredient together in a bowl and add to pan, put beef and stir well. Enjoy!

Chicken Parmesan
So delicious! You need to try this.

Serves: 4

Ingredients

4 boneless and skinless chicken breasts

1/2 cup marinara sauce

4 slices mozzarella cheese

1/2 teaspoon Italian seasonings

1/2 teaspoon garlic powder

1 tablespoon olive oil

Salt and pepper

Directions

1. Add salt, garlic, and pepper to chicken. Add sauce, herbs, and cheese to each chicken breast separately.

2. Heat oil in a skillet and cook chicken breast until cheese melts and brown. Serve!

White Chicken Chili
Well flavored and tasty!

Serves: 12

Ingredients

2 lbs. boneless and skinless chicken breasts, diced

28 oz. chicken stock, low sodium

4 cannellini beans, rinsed

2 cups corn, frozen

3/4 cup low fat Monterey jack cheese, shredded

1 teaspoon ground cumin

1/8 teaspoon cloves, ground

1/8 teaspoon cayenne pepper

1/2 teaspoon chili powder

2 green chili

1 lime, squeezed

1 tablespoon olive oil

3 cloves garlic, grated

1 onion, diced

1 teaspoon salt

Directions

1. Cook onion and chicken in oil on medium heat, put spices, garlic, stock, beans, and cook for about 30 minutes.

2. Put corn, green chili, chili powder, and cook for about 5 minutes and remove from heat. Serve, squeeze lime and put 1 tablespoon cheese in each soup served.

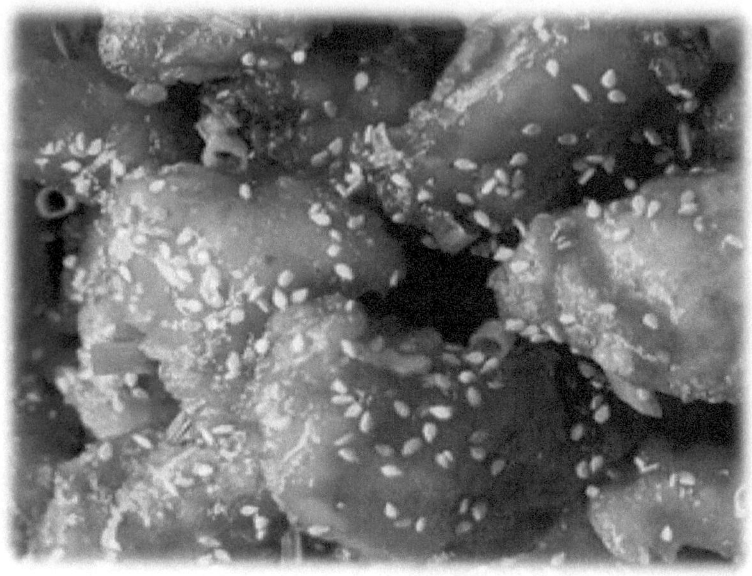

Sesame Chicken

Really healthy and tasty as well!

Serves: 4

Ingredients

1 pound boneless skinless chicken breast, cut

2 tablespoon raw cane sugar

1 teaspoon honey

3 tablespoon soy sauce

1/4 cup white sesame seeds

3 tablespoon olive oil

1/2 teaspoon garlic powder

Black pepper,

Ground cinnamon

Ground ginger

<u>Directions</u>

1. Mix all ingredients together in a bowl except the chicken. Then seasoning chicken with the mixture.

2. Keep in the fridge for about 2 hours. Arrange chicken in a cookie sheet, add a little oil and bake for about 5 minutes at 350 degrees in the oven.

3. Turn to the other side and bake for another 5 minutes. Serve with brown rice or veggies of your choice.

Chicken Croquettes
Very easy to cook!

Serves: 8

<u>Ingredients</u>

4 cups chicken, cooked and shredded

1/4 cup breadcrumbs, seasoned

2 tablespoons poultry seasoning

1 cup cheddar cheese, shredded

2 eggs

1/4 onion, chopped

<u>Directions</u>

1. Add all ingredient together in bowl and refrigerate for about 30 minutes. Cover skillet with cooking spray.

2. Divide mixture into 8 portions and cook for about 5 minutes on each sides. When cheese has melt and crispy, it's ready.

Low-fat Cheeseburger Pie
Really healthy for you!

Serves: 8

Ingredients

1 pound extra lean ground turkey

3/4 cup of Heart Smart Bisquick baking mix

1 cup fat-free cottage cheese

3/4 cup low-fat cheddar cheese, shredded

1 tablespoons Worcestershire sauce

4 slices tomato

1 egg

1/4 cup water

1 clove garlic, chopped

1/2 cup onion, chopped

Directions

1. Mix baking mix and water in bowl, and roll a flat dough like the size of a pie pan.

2. Cook turkey, onion, and garlic to brown. Add sauce and stir.

3. Mix cottage egg and cheese in a bowl. Put dough in a pie pan, put turkey mixture, egg mixture, and tomatoes.

4. Bake for about 40 minutes at 350 degrees and enjoy!

Authentic Mexican Salsa

Sumptuous! Try this.

Serves: 8

Ingredients

1/4 bunch of cilantro

½ teaspoon garlic, minced

½ lemon, squeezed

3 large tomatoes, diced

2 jalapenos, chopped

1 onion, diced

1 teaspoon of salt

Directions

1. Combine all ingredients together and serve. Enjoy!

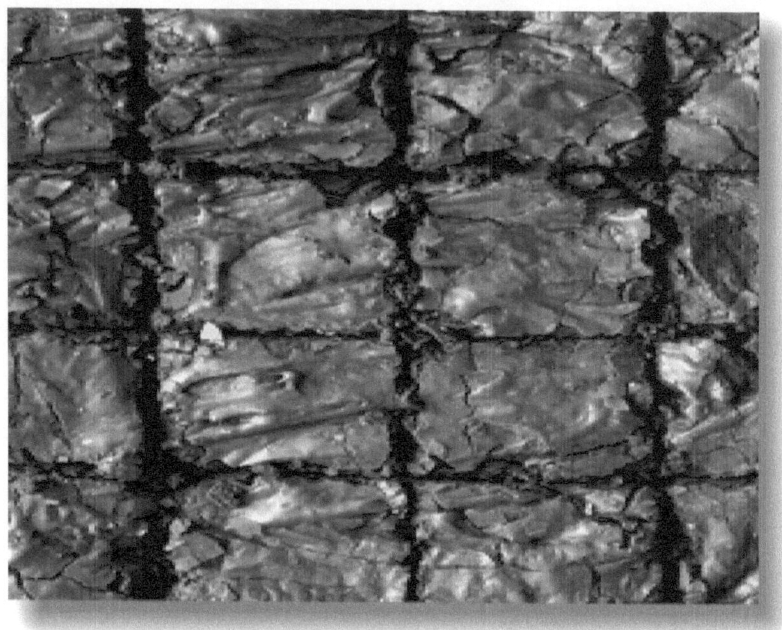

Diet Soda Brownies

Very easy and filling too!

Serves: 12

Ingredients

½ can diet Soda

1 box brownie mix

Directions

1. Mix all together and put to greased pan and bake as stated in the box.

Diet Yellow Cake
Satisfying! Easy to make.

Serves: 18

Ingredients

1 box yellow cake mix

1 can diet soda, white

1 diet mountain dew

Directions

1. Mix all together and bake in 18 muffin cups.

Chocolate Coconut Macaroon Bars
Healthy!

Serves: 6

Ingredients

1 cup Medjool dates, pitted

1 cup almonds, raw

½ teaspoon ground cinnamon

1 teaspoon pure vanilla extract

½ teaspoon cocoa powder

2 tablespoon water

¼ cup almond butter

Salt to taste

Directions

1. Mix all ingredients together except water into a food processor and add a tablespoon of water.

2. Pulse to dough and smooth, add water if needed, meld dough on a cutting board and cut into 6 bars. Enjoy!

Strawberry Blueberry Cherry Kale Ice Pops
Very easy pops and healthy for you!

Serves: 4

Ingredients

2 cups melted frozen fruit mix strawberries,

Blueberries,

Cherries,

Kale

1/4 cup of any fruit juice

Directions

1. Blend fruit mix and add fruit juice. Let it blend smoothly and pour into 4 plastics or paper cups (4 ounce size). Cover with foil.

2. Put pop stick in the center of the cup piercing the foil inside. Refrigerate for about 5 hours and enjoy!

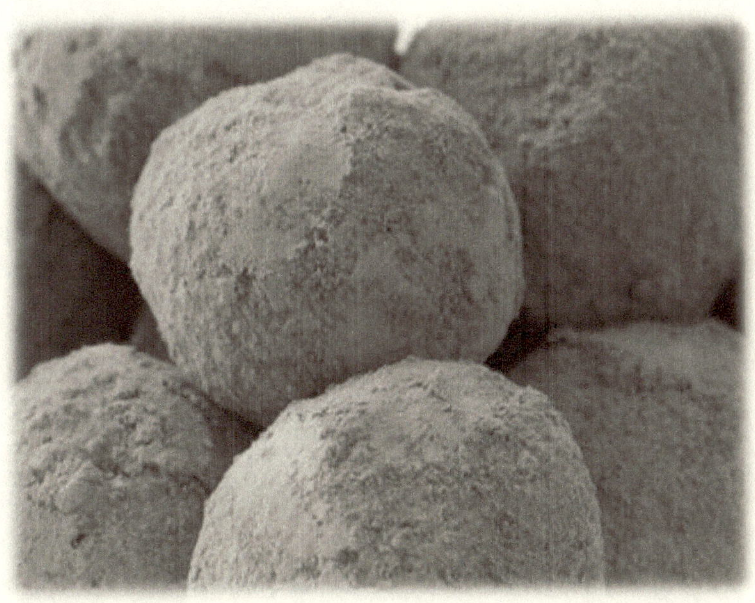

Dark Chocolate Coconut Bites

Just a bite will wow you!

Serves: *18*

Ingredients

2 cups dry coconut

4 tablespoons honey

5 tablespoons coconut oil

1 teaspoon alcohol-free vanilla

4 oz. dark chocolate

Directions

1. Put coconut in a food processor and pulse until smooth like flour. Then pour into a bowl and put honey, vanilla, and coconut.

2. Stir well and use your hand to crush and form 18 ½ balls with the mixture. Put in a cookie sheet lined with parchment paper.

3. Refrigerate for about 30 minutes. Melt 4 oz. dark chocolate over a double-boiler gently until smooth and can be spread.

4. Use two forks to roll each refrigerated balls in the melted chocolate and let it cover the balls round. Place on the lined cookie sheet and refrigerate until the chocolate is hard. Enjoy!

Clean Peach Crumble
Tasty crumble!

Serves: *9*

Ingredients

4 large peaches, diced

3/4 cup old-fashioned oats

2 tablespoon cornstarch

1/4 cup whole wheat flour

2 tablespoon coconut oil

1 ½ teaspoon alcohol-free almond extract

1 teaspoon ground cinnamon

2 tablespoon agave

Directions

1. Mix well almond extract, peaches, pinch of cinnamon and cornstarch. Mix well in another bowl oats, flour, and the cinnamon left.

2. Put peach mixture in a baking dish and sprinkle oats mixture on it. Bake for about 45 minutes at 350°F.

3. Let it cool and enjoy!

Chocolate-Avocado Mousse

Healthy! Try it.

Serves: 3/4

Ingredients

1/2 cup bittersweet chocolate chips

1/2 cup unsweetened cocoa powder

4 ripe avocados, peeled and pitted

1 tablespoon pure vanilla extract

1/2 cup agave

1/3 cup almond milk

1/4 teaspoon salt

Fresh raspberries

Directions

1. Put chips in a bowl and place in a pan with small water on medium heat and simmer for about 3 minutes until chocolate melts.

2. Pulse avocado, chocolate, agave, vanilla, almond milk, cocoa powder and salt in a food processor until smooth

3. Refrigerate for about 3 hours, serve and garnish with fresh raspberries.

Liver-Friendly Pecan Pie Cookies
This is delicious!

Serves: 18

Ingredients

1/3 cup dates, chopped

5 tablespoons pure maple syrup

1/4 teaspoon alcohol-free vanilla extract

1 tablespoon almond milk

1 1/2 cups pecans, chopped

1/4 cup coconut oil

1/8 teaspoon sea salt

2 1/4 cup blanched almond flour, packed

3 tablespoons pure maple syrup

5 tablespoons coconut oil, at room temperature

1 1/2 teaspoons alcohol-free vanilla extract

1/4 teaspoon baking soda

1-2 tablespoons almond milk

1/4 teaspoon sea salt

Directions

1. Put dates in hot water for about 10 minutes. Drain water and set aside. Put almond milk, maple syrup, vanilla, and coconut oil in a sauce pan on medium heat.

2. Remove from heat, blend, add dates and blend until smooth. Set pecan pie filling aside.

3. Mix to dough almond flour, maple syrup, baking soda, vanilla, coconut oil, almond milk, and salt. Roll into balls and put in a cookie sheet.

4. Use a tablespoon to flatten the balls and add the pecan pie filling on each dough and bake for about 14 minutes at 350 degrees. Enjoy when cool!

Healthy Black Bean Brownies
You won't believe the taste! It's delicious.

Serves: 12

Ingredients

1.15oz. can organic black beans, drained

2 tablespoon cocoa powder

2 teaspoon alcohol-free pure vanilla extract

1/2 teaspoon baking powder

1/2 cup pure maple syrup

1/2 cup chocolate chips

1/4 cup coconut oil

1/2 cup quick oats

1/4 teaspoon salt

Directions

1. Pulse until smooth all ingredients in a food processor except chips. Put chips, stir and pour into a pan.

2. Bake for about 18 minutes at 350 degrees. Enjoy when cool.

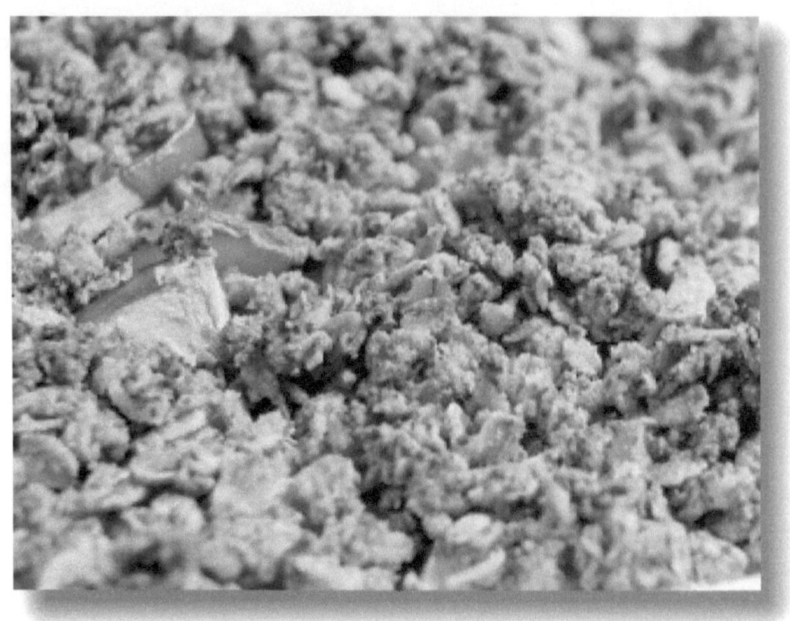

Apple Crumble

Incredibly delicious and chewy for you!

Serves: 6

<u>Ingredients</u>

4 apples, cored, peeled &diced

1/3 cup ground almonds

2 cups quinoa, cooked

1/2 cashews, chopped

2 teaspoons cinnamon

1 teaspoon coconut oil

1 cup flour

Directions

1. Oil the baking dish, put apples in it, mix all ingredients in a bowl, and pour in the baking dish.

2. Bake for about 30 minutes at 350 degrees until brown and apple is soft.

Apple Pie Oatmeal Cookies
This is with a different taste!

Serves: 15

Ingredients

3/4 cup whole wheat flour

1 cup instant oats

1 teaspoon vanilla extract

1 ½ teaspoon baking powder

1 ½ teaspoon ground cinnamon

1 cup red apple, diced

2 tablespoon coconut oil

½ cup honey

1/8 teaspoon salt

1 egg

Directions

1. Mix in a bowl flour, cinnamon, baking powder, and salt. In another mix egg, coconut oil, honey, and vanilla.

2. Combine together the mixtures and sprinkle the apple. Refrigerate for about 30 minutes.

3. Heat at 325°F in the oven and make 15 scoops out of it and bake for about 15 minutes at 325°F.

Mint Chip

Most easy and super delicious!

Serves: 2

Ingredients

2 overripe, frozen bananas, peeled and blended

3 tablespoon broken-up dark chocolate

1teaspoon pure peppermint extract

Pinch of salt

Directions

1. Blend bananas, peppermint extract, and salt. Stir in chocolate and refrigerate until hardened.

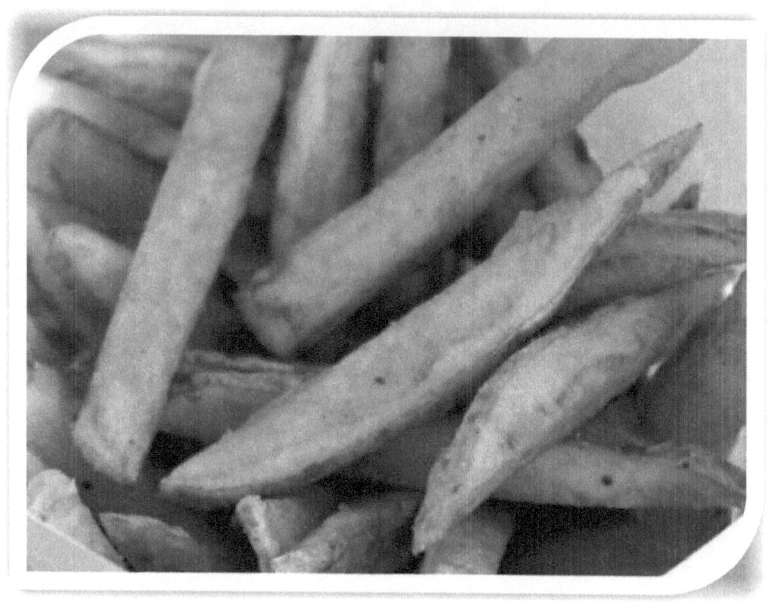

Baked Zucchini Fries

Crispy and chewy! So healthy.

Serves: 6

Ingredients

3 zucchini cut into fries

1/4 cup flour

1/2 cup milk

1 cup breadcrumbs

1/4 teaspoon garlic powder

1/4 cup flour

1/4 teaspoon salt

Directions

1. Mix flour, garlic powder, and salt together. Pour milk and bread crumbs in a separate bowl too.

2. Dip zucchini in flour mixture, again in bread crumbs and in milk, then put in a baking sheet lined with parchment paper.

3. Do that for all the zucchini and bake at 425F for about 20 minutes in the oven. Serve!

Blueberry Energy Bites

So healthy and super easy too!

Serves: 12

Ingredients

1 cup dried blueberries

2 cup raw old-fashioned oats

½ cup almond butter

½ teaspoon cinnamon

1 teaspoon alcohol-free vanilla

½ cup honey

Directions

1. Mix butter, cinnamon, honey, oats, blueberries and vanilla in a bowl.

2. Refrigerate for about 60 minutes until hardened. Form into balls and serve. Enjoy!

Healthier Rice Krispy Treats

This is what you need for snacks any day!

Serves: 16

Ingredients

4 cups Gluten Free, puffed brown rice cereal

1 teaspoon pure vanilla extract

2/3 cup honey

½ cup peanut butter

Salt

Directions

1. Mix all ingredients until combine in a bowl, spread on a baking pan lined with parchment paper and refrigerate for about an hour. Cut and serve.

Crispy Roasted Chickpeas
Yummy!

Serves: 16

Ingredients

2.15-ounce cans of chickpeas, drained

2 tablespoons extra-virgin olive oil

½ teaspoon salt

Directions

1. Spread chickpeas on a baking sheet and refrigerate, put in a paper towels to dry well. Place back on a baking sheet and mix with oil

2. Add salt, mix, spread well, and bake for about 50 minutes at 400°F. When cool, serve.

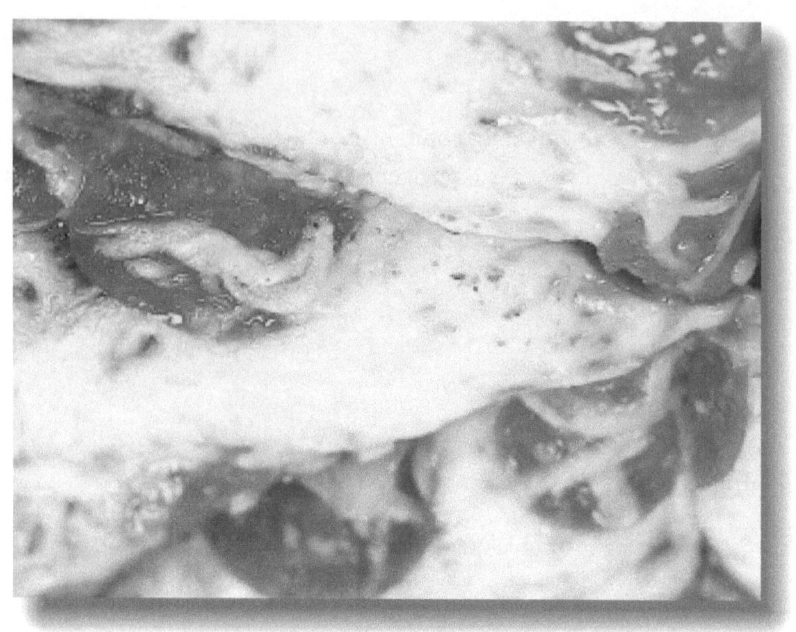

Cauliflower Crust Pizza
This is tasty, you need to make more!

Serves: 6

<u>Ingredients</u>

1 small head cauliflower, chopped

1 1/2 cups shredded low-moisture mozzarella

1/2 cup marinara sauce

1/4 cup fresh basil leaves, torn

1 cup grated Parmesan

1/2 teaspoon dried Italian seasoning

1 clove garlic, minced

1 egg

Olive oil

1/2 teaspoon salt

Freshly ground black pepper

Directions

1. Put a baking sheet upside down in the oven at 475 degrees. Pulse smoothly cauliflower and put in a towel to dry.

2. Put cauliflower in bowl and mix in, parmesan, seasoning, black pepper, egg, garlic and salt.

3. Spread mixture in another baking sheet lined with parchment paper brushed with oil, and slide parchment to the baking sheet in the oven.

4. Bake for about 15 minutes and top with half of mozzarella, sauce, and the second half of mozzarella and bake for another 4 minutes. Garnish with basil, cut and serve.

Almond and Honey-Butter Cookies
The best cookie ever! Try it.

Serves: 3½ dozen

Ingredients

1 cup whole almonds, toasted

1 cup all-purpose flour

1 ¼ cups whole-wheat pastry flour

4 tablespoons unsalted butter, divided

1 teaspoon vanilla extract

3 tablespoons toasted sliced almonds

1 teaspoon baking powder

2/3 cup honey

1/4 cup honey

1/3 cup canola oil

1 large egg

½ teaspoon salt

Directions

1. Pulse almond flour well in a food processor and turn in a bowl, add all-purpose flour, whole-wheat flour, baking powder and salt. Stir well to combine.

2. Beat oil, a little of honey, 3 tablespoons butter, vanilla, and egg in an electric mixer. Beat until well melded.

3. Add flour mixture with honey mixture and combine. Chill for an hour, line with parchment paper and spray with cooking spray two baking sheets.

3. Roll in to ball tablespoons of chilled dough and place in the baking sheets. Use spoons to make lines on cookies.

4. Bake for about 15 minutes at 350 degrees. Mix the remaining honey and butter in a bowl and use in topping the cookies.

Healthy Guacamole

Easy, tasty, and healthy! It's for you.

Serves: 1

Ingredients

3 ripe avocados, cut into half

2 tomatoes, seeded and diced

3 tablespoons fresh cilantro, chopped

4 garlic cloves, minced

1 lime, juiced

½ cup onion, diced

1 teaspoon salt

Directions

1. Scoop out the flesh from avocado, add lime, tomatoes, cilantro, cayenne pepper, onion, garlic and salt

2. Chill or serve immediately as desired.

Local Bean and Mango Salsa

Best meal for you! Snack it.

Serves: 1

Ingredients

1 mango, peeled and diced

1 cup of dried beans, soaked overnight, and boiled

2 limes, juiced

½ jalapeno, flesh removed, seeded and diced

¼ cup cilantro, chopped

1 large tomatoes, seeded and diced

2 tablespoons organic olive oil

1 onion, diced

Directions

1. Add all ingredients together in a bowl and toss. Put salt and pepper to taste. Enjoy salsa with roasted corn!

Pico de Gallo

Fantastic recipe with a delicious taste!

Serves: 1

<u>Ingredients</u>

3 jalapenos, skinned, seeded and chopped

10vine tomatoes, diced

1 lime, juiced

1 onion, diced

1½ cups fresh cilantro, chopped

¼ teaspoon salt

<u>Directions</u>

1. Mix in a bowl onions, cilantro, tomatoes, lime, and jalapeno to combine. Add salt to taste and enjoy with chips or tortillas.

Cashew-Less Vegan Queso Dip

Dip to always look for, anytime!

Serves: 1

Ingredients

6 whole wheat pitas, cut in half and 8 wedges

1 teaspoon chili powder

1 teaspoon garlic powder

2 teaspoons olive oil

Salt

Directions

1. Place pitas on a baking sheet without overlapping, and brush with oil. Sprinkle with salt, chili and garlic powder.

2. Bake for about 8 minutes until lightly golden at 400°F. Enjoy!

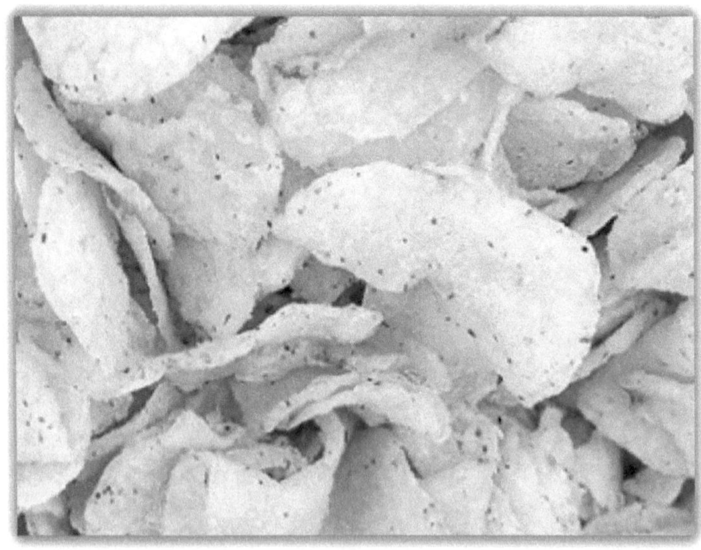

Microwave Potato Chips

Tasty and crunchy for you!

Serves: 2

Ingredients

1 medium russet potato, peeled and sliced thinly

Seasoning

Salt

Directions

1. Put potatoes on a glass paper and sprinkle seasoning and salt.

2. Microwave for about 5 minutes on high until potatoes are brown light.

Chili Popcorn

Super tasty popcorn to always remember! You should try this.

Serves: 4

Ingredients

1 quart popcorn, popped

1/4 teaspoon ground cumin

1 ¼ teaspoons chili powder

½ tablespoon margarine, melted

Garlic powder

Directions

1. Mix margarine with popcorn to combine, add cumin, garlic and chili powder. Enjoy!

SALAD RECIPES

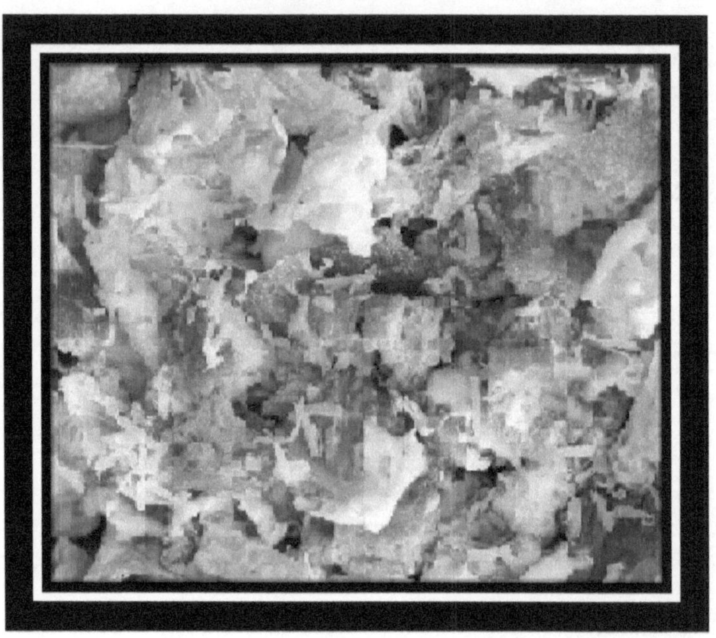

Cabbage Slaw

Super easy! This is just best for you.

Serves: 4

Ingredients

1 ½ cups green cabbage, sliced

2 cups Napa cabbage, sliced

½ cup red cabbage, thinly sliced

1 teaspoon fresh ginger root, grated

2 tablespoons rice wine vinegar

3 tablespoons orange marmalade

1 tablespoon fresh chives, chopped

Directions

1. Combine cabbage and chives, combine ginger, vinegar and marmalade, add to cabbage mixture. Toss and enjoy!

Liver-Friendly Potato Salad

Yummy! This tastes so well.

Serves: 8

Ingredients

4 large potatoes, cubed and steamed

2 teaspoons mustard powder

2 tablespoons of fresh parsley

2 cloves garlic, minced

½ cup extra virgin olive oil

½ cup lemon juice

1 red onion, chopped

1 ½ teaspoon sea salt

Directions

1. Add mustard powder, lemon juice, and salt to a bowl and combine. Add mixture to potatoes, put garlic and onion, stir gently and chill.

2. When chilled put parsley and oil, stir and serve.

California Roll in a Bowl

This is delicious, you should try it.

Serves: 4

Ingredients

1 cup brown rice, cooked

8 oz. cooked shrimp, chopped

1 English cucumber, seedless and sliced

1 romaine lettuce, chopped

3 tablespoon rice wine vinegar

1 tablespoon light soy sauce

½ teaspoon wasabi powder

3 tablespoon pickled ginger, chopped

1 large sheet nori seaweed, toasted and broken

1 ripe avocado, diced

1 teaspoon sesame seeds

1 carrot, grated

Directions

1. Mix soy sauce, rice wine vinegar, and wasabi powder together to combine to make dressing. Set aside.

2. Share lettuce into four plates, top each plate with avocado, carrot, crab meat, ginger, and cucumber.

3. Top each plates with dressing, sesame seeds and nori. Enjoy!

Israeli Salad

The best so far for you!

Serves: 8

Ingredients

1 medium cucumber, peeled and chopped

3 medium tomatoes, chopped

1 bell pepper, desired color

2 tablespoon lemon juice

1 teaspoon fresh ground pepper

3 tablespoon extra-virgin olive oil

1 teaspoon salt

Directions

1. Combine all ingredients together and enjoy!

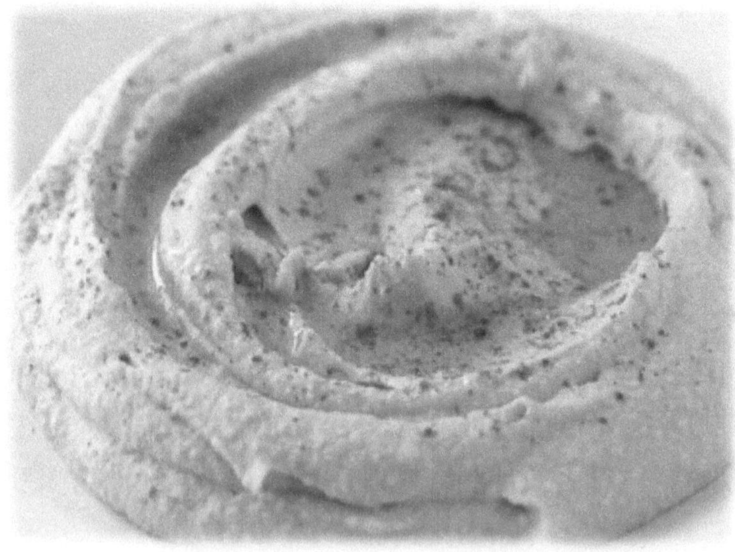

Hummus
This dip is super healthy!

Serves: 14

Ingredients

2.15 ounce cans of chickpeas, rinsed

1 tablespoon tahini

2 clove of garlic, grated

1 tablespoon olive oil

Sweet paprika

Directions

1. Pulse chickpeas, garlic, tahini, oil, and a little water in a food processor until smooth and thick. Top with paprika and enjoy with pita bread if desired or veggies.

Pasta and Veggies Salad
So fresh and really tasty!

Serves: 8

Ingredients

13.25 oz. of whole grain pasta

4 cups fresh broccoli, pieces

¾ cup balsamic vinaigrette salad dressing

3 tablespoons fresh parsley, chopped

1 tablespoon lemon pepper

1 sweet red bell pepper, sliced

6 fresh basil leaves, sliced thin

4 teaspoons lemon juice, fresh

16 oz. whole black olives, drained (1can)

¼ red Onion, sliced

Directions

1. Cook pasta according to the direction, drain and add all ingredient except lemon pepper. Stir and chill for about 2 hours. Serve and enjoy with lemon pepper.

Salad with Chicken and Berries
Delicious!

Serves: 4

Ingredients

12 ounces rotisserie chicken breast, skinless, boneless and sliced

4 cups romaine lettuce, torn

2 cups strawberries, quartered

1 cup fresh blueberries

2 tablespoons red wine vinegar

1/8 teaspoon freshly ground black pepper

2 tablespoons extra-virgin olive oil

4 cups arugula

1/3 cup red onion, sliced

1/8 teaspoon salt

<u>Directions</u>

1. Mix red water, wine vinegar, black pepper and salt in a small bowl for dressing. Combine strawberries, romaine, blueberries, arugula, and onions for salad. Toss, share into four, and dress.

Massaged Kale Salad

Super tasty!

Serves: 4

<u>Ingredients</u>

1 large bunch kale, stalk removed and sliced

2 tablespoons toasted pumpkin seeds

2 teaspoons honey

1 fresh mango, diced

1 lemon, juiced

¼ extra-virgin olive oil

Salt

Freshly ground black pepper

<u>Directions</u>

1. Put kale, half of lemon juice, and salt in a bowl and massage. Add oil and massage.

2. Combine in another bowl honey, ground black pepper, and remaining lemon juice for dressing. Add salt to taste.

3. Put dressing in kale and top with mango and pumpkin seeds.

Greek Salad

Delicious and healthy salad for you!

Serves: 4

Ingredients

1 English cucumber, seeded, and sliced

1 yellow bell pepper, seeded and diced

1 pint grape tomatoes, halved

1 orange bell pepper, seeded and diced

½ teaspoon Dijon mustard

¼ cup red wine vinegar

½ cup black olives, pitted

½ teaspoon freshly ground black pepper

½ red onion, sliced

½ cup black olives, pitted

2 cloves garlic, minced

1 teaspoon dried oregano

½ cup good olive oil

Directions

1. Put red onions, cucumber, and tomatoes in a bowl, and combine. In another bowl combine vinegar, oregano, garlic, oil, oregano, mustard, salt and pepper for dressing.

2. Add dressing to vegetables and toss. Enjoy!

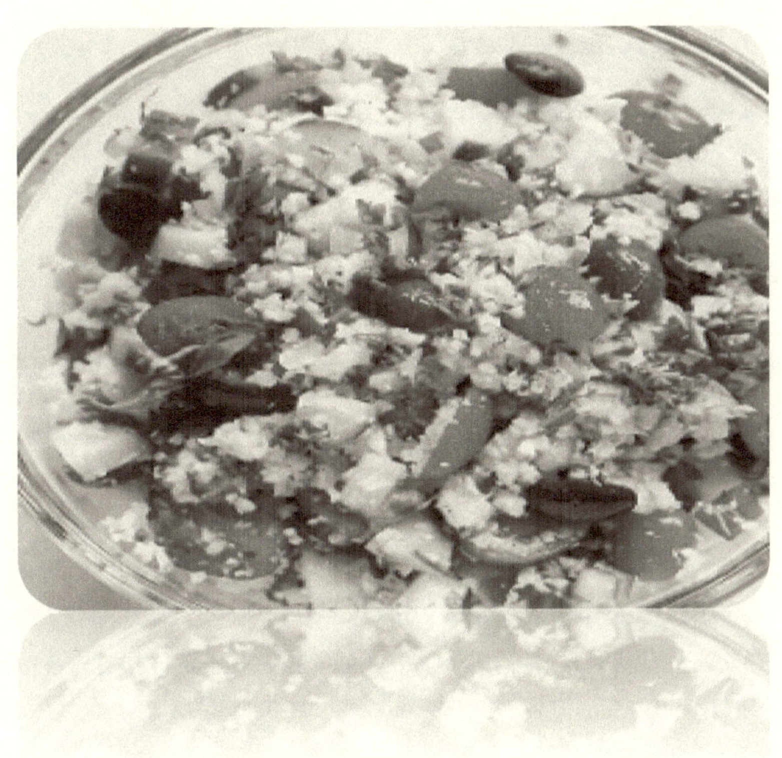

Detox Salad

Full of flavor and nutritious!

Serves: 4

Ingredients

½ medium sized red cabbage, shredded

2 tablespoon fresh parsley, chopped

2 tablespoon fresh squeezed lemon juice

3 tablespoon pine nuts, toasted

1 tablespoon pumpkin seeds

2 tablespoon sunflower seeds

2 tablespoon flax seed

2 teaspoon grated ginger root

2 apples, cored and sliced

2 celery sticks, sliced

1 teaspoon honey

3 carrots, grated

4 tablespoon olive oil

Directions

1. Combine red cabbage, carrots, parsley, apples, celery sticks, pine nuts, pumpkin seeds, sunflower seeds, and flax seed together in a bowl for salad.

2. Combine in another bowl ginger root, honey, squeezed lemon juice, and olive oil for dressing. Put over salad and enjoy!

Easy Watermelon and Feta Salad
Super easy to make! Best for you.

Serves: 8

Ingredients

2 tablespoons feta cheese, crumbled

½ cup fat-free Greek yogurt

6 cups seedless watermelon, cubed

½ bunch cilantro, chopped

2 stalks celery, sliced

¼ teaspoon black pepper

¼ teaspoon black pepper

1 teaspoon lemon juice

1 tablespoon lime juice

1 red onion, sliced

Directions

1. Combine watermelon, celery, onion, black pepper, and feta cheese for salad.

2. Combine lemon juice, lime juice, cilantro, yogurt, and black pepper for dressing, mix with salad and enjoy!

Cucumber Salad with Vinegar and Onion
You will enjoy this salad!

Serves: 6

Ingredients

5 cucumbers, peel and sliced

½ cup water

½ cup white vinegar

1 red onion, sliced

Salt and pepper

Directions

1. Mix cucumber and onions to combine. Combine vinegar, salt, pepper, and water in another bowl for dressing. Enjoy!

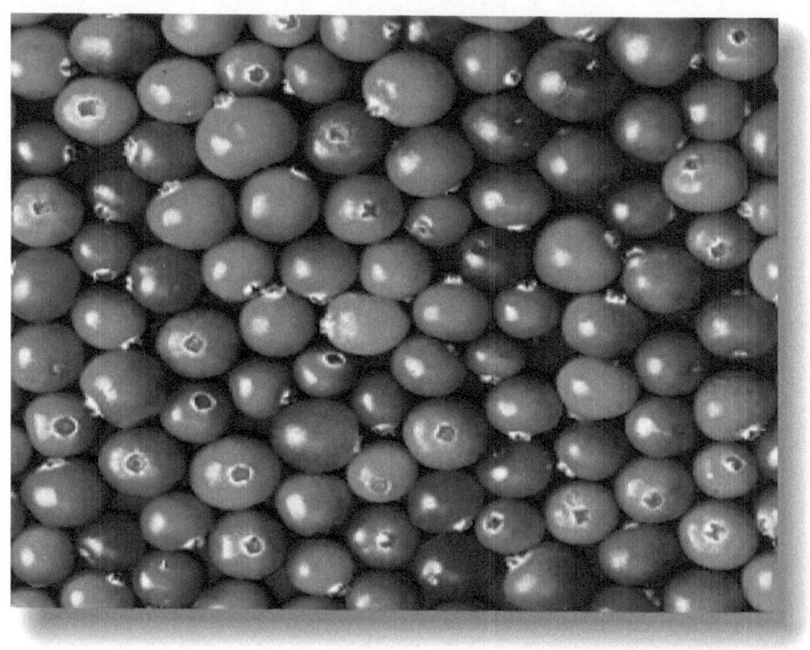

Cranberry Juice

Healthy and tasty juice for you only!

Serves: 1

Ingredients

8 ounce light cranberry juice

¾ cup orange juice

¼ cup lemon juice

¼ teaspoon ground nutmeg

4 tablespoon ground flax seeds

¼ teaspoon ground ginger

½ teaspoon ground cinnamon

Water

Directions

1. Boil cinnamon, nutmeg, cranberry juice, and water in a pot, when cool, add ginger, lemon and orange juice. Refrigerate. Put flax seed when ready to serve.

Christmas Punch

The taste makes the difference! You should taste this.

Serves: 16

Ingredients

64 oz. cranberry juice

2 liters diet sprite zero

2 limes, juiced

Ice

Directions

1. Mix juice, sprite, and lime in a bowl. Add any fruit of your choice and refrigerate. Enjoy with ice.

Sparkling Pomegranate Punch

Tasty punch for you!

Serves: 9

Ingredients

3 cups orange juice

3 cups diet lemon-lime soda

3 cups pomegranate juice

Directions

1. Combine all together and enjoy!

Homemade Oat Milk
Best family choice!

Serves: 8

Ingredients

1 cup gluten-free rolled oats

1 tablespoon maple syrup

Water

Salt

Directions

1. Blend all ingredients smoothly, sieve and use a towel to strain milk from the chaff. Shake and enjoy!

Watermelon, Pineapple, Turmeric Smoothie
Tasty and healthy for you!

Serves: 2

Ingredients

2 cups frozen watermelon, cubed

1 orange, peeled, seeded

2 cups frozen pineapple, cubed

1 ½ cups coconut water, frozen

2 teaspoons turmeric, grated

½ cup coconut milk

1 teaspoon ginger, grated

Directions

1. Blend all ingredients and enjoy!

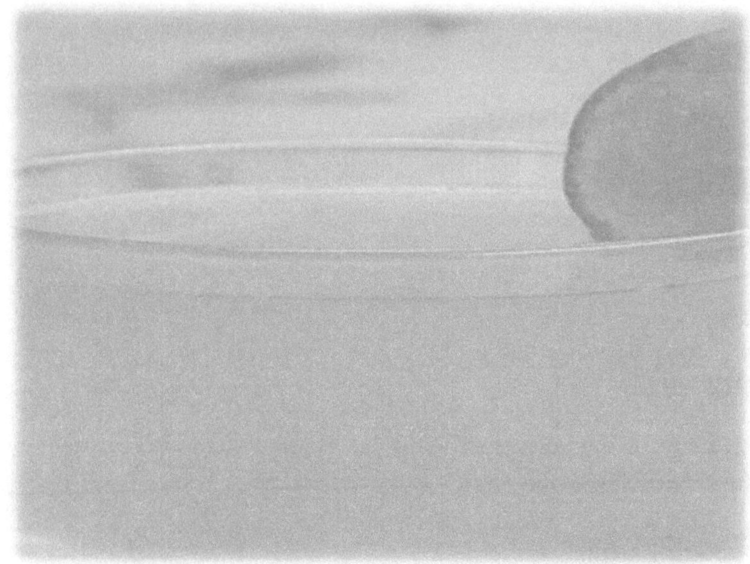

Ginger Lemonade

Full of nutrient and tasty!

Serves: 8

Ingredients

2 tablespoons ginger root, peeled and grated

4 large strips of lemon peel

2 medium sprigs fresh rosemary

1/3 cup honey

4 lemons, juiced

Directions

1. Bring to boil lemon peels, rosemary and ginger. Sieve, add 6 cups of cold water, honey and lemon juice to juice. Serve with ice.

Homemade Water Kefir Soda

This soda is super delicious!

Serves: 8

Ingredients

2liters temperature filtered water

½ water kefir grains

1 Organic grape juice

½ Organic brown sugar

Directions

1. Boil 1 cup filtered water and brown sugar. Let it cool and set aside. Mix ½ cup water kefir grains and 1 liter filtered water in a jar.

2. Add cooled brown sugar to the mixture of grains and water. Add the remaining water and cover jar to ferment for about 48 hours.

3. When fermented divide into four jars, and add ¼ organic grape juice into each jar and strain with a clean kitchen towel. Put into 8cup of glass and enjoy!

Mojito Mock Tail

This will help you forget cocktail!

Serves: 8

Ingredients

3 lime slices

11 fresh mint leaves

1 tablespoon honey

6 ounces soda water

Directions

1. Mix lime and mint leaves together, crush to release flavor, and put honey, soda water and ice. Enjoy!

Turmeric Tea – Golden Milk

Creamy and super taste! You will surely enjoy this.

Serves: 4

Ingredients

2 cups of coconut milk, or any desired milk

¼ teaspoon ground ginger powder

½ teaspoon cinnamon

1 teaspoon raw honey

1 teaspoon turmeric

Black pepper

Directions

1. Blend all ingredients and heat for about 3 minutes. Drink hot.

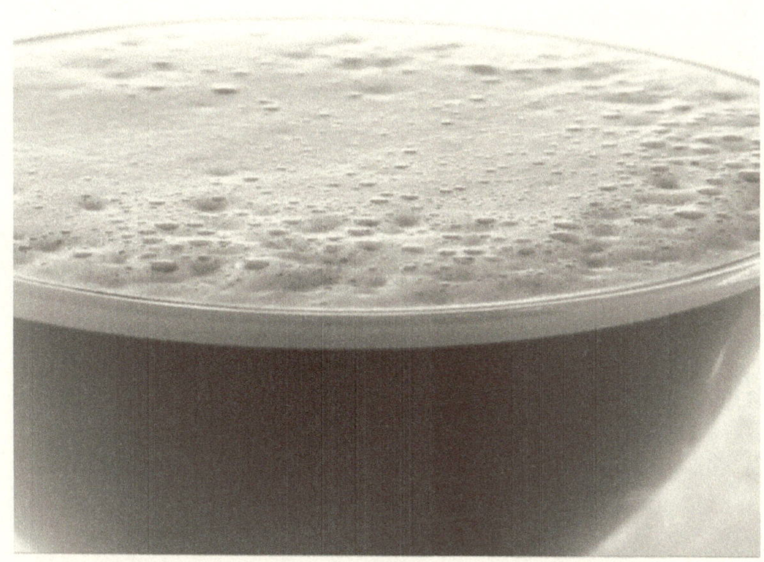

Healthy Shamrock Shake

Tasty shake you will definitely enjoy!

Serves: 2

Ingredients

2 cups vanilla frozen yogurt

½ teaspoon alcohol-free mint extract

1 ½ cups vanilla almond milk

1 scoop Ultra-nourish

Directions

1. Blend smoothly all ingredients and enjoy with ice.

Delicious Iced Coffee
You will enjoy this coffee!

Serves: 24

Ingredients

1 pound ground coffee

8 quarts cold water, (32 cups)

Ice

Directions

1. Mix coffee with water and soak for about eight hours, strain and refrigerate. Enjoy with ice and add milk if desired!

Healthy Homemade Pumpkin Spice Latte
This is different! You need it.

Serves: 1

Ingredients

3 tablespoons pumpkin puree

½ cup unsweetened vanilla almond milk

1 teaspoon pumpkin pie spice

8 ounces fresh-brewed coffee

3 drops of liquid stevia

½ teaspoon alcohol-free vanilla

Cinnamon

<u>**Directions**</u>

1. Cook pumpkin and almond milk, add spices, vanilla, and sweetener. Blend until foamy, put coffee in a cut and add milk mixture. Sprinkle cinnamon.